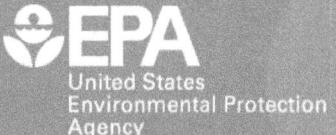

United States
Environmental Protection
Agency

EPA 600/R-11/054 | June 2011 | www.epa.gov/ord

I0494222

Planning for an Emergency
Drinking Water Supply

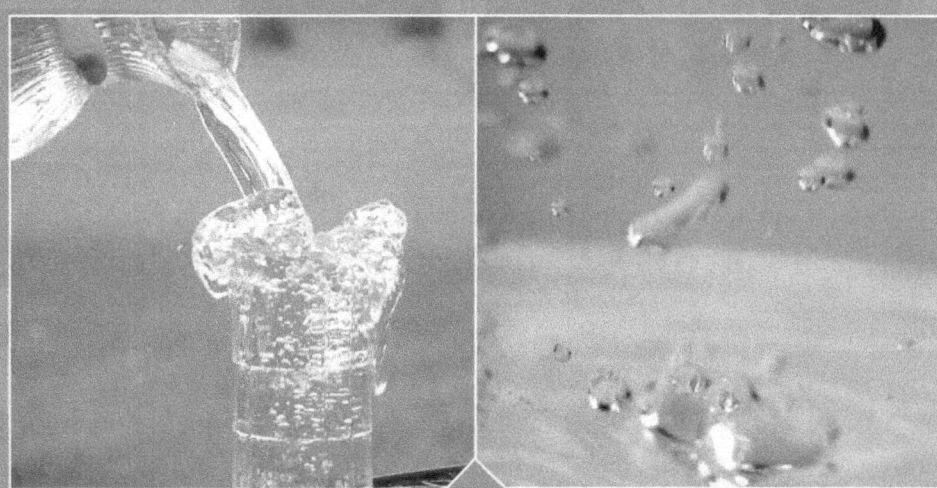

Office of Research and Development
National Homeland Security Research Center

Planning for an Emergency Drinking Water Supply

**Prepared for U.S. Environmental Protection Agency's
National Homeland Security Research Center by
American Water Works Association and CDM**

June 2011

Table of Contents

List of Tables

List of Figures

Acknowledgements

Funding for this project was provided by U.S. Environmental Protection Agency (EPA) under order number EP08C000294 and the American Water Works Association (AWWA) Water Industry Technical Action Fund Project #516.

Project Team

EPA Office of Research and Development, National Homeland Security Research Center

Steve Clark, Project Officer

American Water Works Association

Kevin M. Morley, Security & Preparedness Program Manager

CDM

Phillippe Daniel, Vice President and Project Manager

Craig von Bargen, Vice President and Technical Reviewer

Paula Kulis, Engineer

Julie Hinchcliff, Report

Juan Tijero, Graphics

Project Steering Committee

Robert Babcock, Michigan Department of Environmental Quality

Mike Boufis, Bethpage Water District, New York

Ted Corrigan, Des Moines Water, Iowa

Steve Dennis, Alameda County Water District, California

George Hoke, Fairfax Water Authority, Virginia

Workshop Participants and Peer Review

We gratefully acknowledge the time and input received by those who attended workshops held in Washington, D.C. (June 2009, January 2010, and June 2010), Los Angeles (September 2009) and Atlanta (December 2009).

Peer review was provided by Jim Wheeler, OWM, OW, Kevin Garrahan NHSRC, ORD and Nushat Thomas WSD, OW

Workshop Attendees

Name	Affiliation
Washington, D.C. – June 2009	
Peter Gross	Aeromix
Kevin Morley	American Water Works Association
Phillippe Daniel	CDM
Tim Ruckman	Department of the Army – Fort Lee (NJ)
David Gragan	District of Columbia
Stephen Clark	EPA – National Homeland Security Research Center
Kevin Tingley	EPA – Water Security Division
Jennifer Rosenberger	Federal Emergency Management Agency (FEMA) – Disaster Operations
Sarah Solli	General Electric
Kyaw Moe	MECO
David Dise	Montgomery County (MD)
Chantel Freidrich	Norit
Mike Delao	Norit
Bruce Bartley	NSF International
Peter Takach	Pall Corporation
Holmes Walters	U.S. Army Corp of Engineers
Los Angeles – September 2009	
Steve Dennis	Alameda County Water District (CA)
Michael Kleiner	American Red Cross – Los Angeles Chapter
Kevin Morley	American Water Works Association
Joe Crisologo	California Department of Public Health
Mark Bassett	California Office of Emergency Services
Phillippe Daniel	CDM
Paula Kulis	CDM
Ted Corrigan	Des Moines Water Works
Mike Ambrose	East Bay Municipal Utility District (CA)
Gary Sturdivan	East Valley Water District (CA)
Steve Clark	EPA – National Homeland Security Research Center
George Hoke	Fairfax Water (VA)
Bob Vincent	Florida Department of Health
Pankaj Parekh	Los Angeles Department of Water & Power
Karen Irion	Louisiana Department of Health and Hospitals
Nick Catrantzos	Metropolitan Water District of Southern California
Shane Chapman	Metropolitan Water District of Southern California
Kelly Hubbard	Orange County Water District (CA)
Robert Alexander	Tennessee Division of Water Pollution Control

Atlanta – December 2009	
Kevin Morley	American Water Works Association
Scott Borman	Benton/Washington Regional Public Water Authority (AR)
Phillippe Daniel	CDM
Jay Watson	Centers for Disease Control
Mark D. Miller	Centers for Disease Control
Mark Austin	Centers for Disease Control
Patti Lamb	Charlotte-Mecklenberg Utilities (NC)
Joe Ramos	City of Atlanta (GA)
Lance Houser	City of Logan (UT)
Ray Riordan	City of San Ramon (CA)
Steve Clark	EPA – National Homeland Security Research Center
Nushat Thomas	EPA – Water Security Division
George Hoke	Fairfax Water (VA)
Brad Addison	Georgia Department of Natural Resources
Sandy Smith	Gwinnett County (GA)
John Smart	Human Health Services
Scott Kelly	JEA (FL)
Robert Babcock	Michigan Department of Environmental Quality
Kim Ketterhagen	Minnesota Department of Public Safety
William "Bill" Morris	New York City Department of Environmental Protection
Mark S. Roupas	Office of the Assistant Secretary of Defense
Washington, D.C. – January 2010	
Darrell Osterhoudt	Association of State Drinking Water Administrators
Kevin Morley	American Water Works Association
Phillippe Daniel	CDM
Stephen Clark	EPA – National Homeland Security Research Center
Kim Fox	EPA – National Homeland Security Research Center
Peter Jutro	EPA – National Homeland Security Research Center
Brendlyn Faison	EPA – Office of Wetlands, Oceans, and Watersheds
Nushat Thomas	EPA – Water Security Division
George Gray	Gray & Associates
Joseph Cotruvo	JAC Associates
Cliff McLellan	NSF International
Jennifer Sass	Natural Resources Defense Council
Steven Richards	Department of the Army - Public Health Command
Todd Richards	Department of the Army - Public Health Command

Washington, D.C. – June 2010	
Omar Abou-Samra	American Red Cross
Kevin Morley	American Water Works Association
Phillippe Daniel	CDM
Stephen Clark	EPA – National Homeland Security Research Center
Tom Kirsch	John Hopkins University
Shelly Shafer	U.S. Army Corp of Engineers
Bill Irwin	U.S. Army Corp of Engineers
Spencer Shardasky	U.S. Army Corp of Engineers (Intern)
Trevor White	U.S. Agency for International Development (USAID) - Office of Foreign Disaster Assistance

List of Acronyms

ASPHER	Assistant Secretary for Public Health Emergency Preparedness
AWWA	American Water Works Association
CDC	Centers for Disease Control and Prevention
DHS	Department of Homeland Security
DOD	Department of Defense
EDWP	Emergency drinking water plan
EOC	Emergency operations center
EPA	Environmental Protection Agency
EPCRA	Emergency Planning and Community Right-to-Know Act
ERP	Emergency response plan
ERT	EPA Environmental Response Team
ESF	Emergency support function
FEMA	Federal Emergency Management Agency
ICS	Incident Command System
JFO	Joint Field Office
LEPC	Local Emergency Planning Committee
MRE	Meals Ready-to-Eat
NGO	Non-Governmental Organization
NIMS	National Incident Management System
NHSRC	National Homeland Security Research Center
NLE	National level exercise
NRF	National Response Framework
POD	Point of distribution
RISC	Regional Interagency Steering Committee
SDWA	Safe Drinking Water Act
SERC	State Emergency Response Commissions
USACE	U.S. Army Corps of Engineers
USAID	U.S. Agency for International Development
WARN	Water and Wastewater Emergency Response Network

Disclaimer

The preparation and publication of this document has been funded by the U.S. Environmental Protection Agency (EPA) under contract number EP08C000294 and the American Water Works Association Water Industry Technical Action Fund Project #516. It has been subjected to the Agency's peer and administrative review and has been approved for publication as an EPA document. Note that approval does not signify that the contents necessarily reflect the views of the Agency. Mention of trade names or commercial products does not constitute endorsement or recommendation for use.

Introduction

Five workshops were convened with about sixty technical experts to review alternative means of providing drinking water in the event of destruction, impairment, or contamination of the public water supply. Various scenarios were assumed, such as destruction or impairment of the water infrastructure by a powerful earthquake and contamination events requiring alternate supplies of drinking water. The term "emergency water supply" will be used instead of the equivalent terms "alternative water supply/sources" throughout this report. Based on the severity of an incident, all levels of government (local, state and federal), as well as non-governmental organizations (NGOs), like the Red Cross, may become involved.

The workshops identified the importance of the development of an emergency drinking water plan by a local water utility, even though, during the actual emergency, other entities (e.g., State National Guard) may be tasked with implementing that plan. The water utility could use this report to assist in developing its plan, i.e., to assemble a group consisting of the Local Emergency Planning Committee (LEPC), NGOs, and state officials to determine appropriate roles and to write a plan for their community. The U.S. EPA strongly encourages utilities to regularly review and update their vulnerability assessments and emergency response plans. The emergency drinking water planning could be viewed as a component of the emergency response plan updates done by the water utility.

Note: This document addresses the supply of drinking water after a disaster. While hygiene and sanitation issues are not addressed herein, they are public health priorities and should be included in emergency planning.

1. Purpose

Provision of emergency water supply involves collaboration and partnership between various levels of government. Although this document is not guidance as to how to comply with any particular law, the following is a helpful review of the roles and responsibilities among various levels of government regarding emergency water supplies. Relevant federal legislative language pertaining to each level (federal, state, and local) is cited herein. The discussion highlights the importance Congress has placed on emergency water supply planning.

Federal -- The Safe Drinking Water Act (SDWA) was amended by the Public Health Security and Bioterrorism Preparedness and Response Act of 2002 (Bioterrorism Act) to address emergency water supplies. The Bioterrorism Act directs EPA to conduct "a review of the methods and means by which alternative supplies of drinking water could be provided in the event of destruction, impairment or contamination of public water systems" (42 U.S.C. 300i-4 (b) .).

The Bioterrorism Act specifies actions that Community Water Supplies and EPA must take to improve the security of the Nation's drinking water infrastructure. This document expands on the discussion in EPA's 2004 guidance for small and medium community water systems (EPA 2004). [1] In addition, it provides more detail on emergency water supply planning for all system sizes, but especially large metropolitan water systems, where planning is more critical due to volume considerations.

Executive Order 12656, dated November 18, 1988, requires the EPA Administrator to take lead responsibility to "develop, in coordination with the Secretary of Defense, plans to assure the provision of potable water supplies to meet community needs under national security emergency conditions, including claimancy for materials and equipment for public water systems." This document covers all instances where emergency water supply is needed, including as a result of natural disasters and national security emergencies.

State -- The responsibilities of state primacy agencies are specified in 42 U.S.C. 300g–2, which provides, in part: "A State has primary enforcement responsibility for public water systems during any period for which the Administrator determines . . . that such State . . . has adopted and can implement an adequate plan for the provision of safe drinking water under emergency circumstances including earthquakes, floods, hurricanes, and other natural disasters, as appropriate" (42 U.S.C. 300g-2(a)(5)).

Typically state agencies are able to render assistance to smaller systems but they may not have the resources to handle large system or regional outages. For large disasters, states typically seek support under provisions of the Robert T. Stafford Disaster Relief and Emergency Assistance Act, 42 U.S.C. 5121-5207 (the "Stafford Act"), which allows federal agencies to provide assistance such as bottled water and public works engineering. The Stafford Act allows a state governor to request assistance through the

---

[1] Element 5 of EPA's 2004 guidance (listed here) provides information on utility selection of alternate water sources: EPA. (2004). "Emergency Response Plan Guidance for Small and Medium Community Water Supply Systems to Comply with the Public Health Security and Bioterrorism Preparedness and Response Act of 2002" U.S. EPA Office of Water (4601M), EPA 816-R-04-002 April 7, 2004. Accessed February 14, 2011. http://www.epa.gov/safewater/watersecurity/pubs/small_medium_ERP_guidance040704.pdf

local disaster field office. State primacy agencies should be familiar with request procedures, and they should incorporate into their planning the level of assistance they are able to provide and when federal supplemental assistance would be required.

Utility -- The responsibilities of drinking water utilities are specified in 42 U.S.C. 300i-2, which provides, in part: "Each community water system serving a population greater than 3,300 shall prepare or revise, where necessary, an emergency response plan that incorporates the results of vulnerability assessments that have been completed . . . The emergency response plan shall include, but not be limited to, plans, procedures, and identification of equipment that can be implemented or utilized in the event of a terrorist or other intentional attack on the public water system. The emergency response plan shall also include actions, procedures, and identification of equipment which can obviate or significantly lessen the impact of terrorist attacks or other intentional actions on the public health and *the safety and supply of drinking water provided to communities and individuals.* Community water systems shall, to the extent possible, coordinate with existing Local Emergency Planning Committees established under the Emergency Planning and Community Right-to-Know Act (42 U.S.C. 11001 et seq.) when preparing or revising an emergency response plan under this subsection" (42 U.S.C. 300i-2(b) (emphasis added).

The statutory language encourages the inclusion of drinking water supply issues in the emergency planning process as utilities coordinate with Local Emergency Planning Committees (LEPCs) to mitigate the impact. The need for collaboration and shared responsibility by many partners to ensure an adequate potable water supply in the aftermath of an event is a point that will be continuously highlighted throughout this document.

2. Summary

The review of legislative language covering emergency water supply planning demonstrates that all levels of government have some responsibility for emergency water supply planning. All government entities and others responsible for emergency water supplies should coordinate roles, identify approaches, and estimate resources. Preplanning leads to more effective and efficient operations under emergency conditions. This document covers the technical details of this planning; Section 9 presents key workshop findings.

The principal findings are:

1. There are several options for supplying potable water in an emergency. These include water supplied via interconnections with neighboring water utilities, bottled water supplied locally or regionally (a common federal response), and locally produced water. Locally produced water can be obtained by packaging pre-treated water, by using mobile treatment units to inject water into the existing distribution system, or by using mobile treatment in conjunction with water packaging or water tap distribution.

2. Utilities should develop an emergency drinking water plan that considers

   a. the various types of maximum credible events to which they are vulnerable [Note: A maximum credible event is one that can reasonably be expected to occur but not in combination with unlikely coincidence, such as an earthquake and hurricane impacting South Carolina simultaneously. What event type would cause the most damage and has some reasonable likelihood of happening?];

   b. the number of people potentially affected and the associated duration for a maximum credible event;

   c. the point at which the local capacity to respond adequately would be exhausted;

   d. the potable water alternatives that are the most feasible for the maximum credible event;

   e. what resources would be needed from others, including regional, state or federal agencies;

   f. the process for communicating these resource requests to the various emergency service agencies; and

   g. how to implement the delivery of needed resources.

3. All planning partners would benefit from a state-level aggregation of the resources gaps identified at local levels. Understanding the aggregated state-level resource gap enables planners to include additional sources as a part of the contingency plan. (See Section 9 for a more detailed discussion of relevant the findings.)

3. Background for this Planning Document

Emergency response efficiency depends on the preparation that has occurred before a disaster. An emergency drinking water plan (EDWP) can be developed in four steps:

1. Assess vulnerability and the potential scale of outage with respect to events, likelihood, and consequences.

Planning requires that utilities identify the events to which their specific utility is vulnerable. They should assess both the likelihood and potential impacts on basic infrastructure and on water distribution operations. The scope and scale of a water outage will vary according to the severity of the event and the condition of a given water system.

2. Determine target levels of service post-event (quantity and quality) based on timing following the onset of the event (i.e., within the first 3 days, 10 days, 21 days). Recommendation is to start with 3 gallons per person per day at a level that is acceptable for human consumption.

3. Analyze alternative drinking water sources and develop a detailed implementation plan.

4. Implement plan - Pre-event, Post-event

The third step of this process is the principal focus of this document. Utilities are charged with emergency response planning, though not necessarily implementation. In a large-scale emergency, local resources would likely be overwhelmed and outside assistance for the procurement and distribution of emergency drinking water would be required. In that case, utilities would have to focus their own resources on restoring service.

An EDWP should address issues ranging from water transport to coordination of the various response partners. It is essential that resource availability is confirmed and that there is no double-counting (i.e., multiple agencies relying on the same resources).

Major Inputs for Developing This Guide
• Literature review
• Consultation with local, state and federal agencies
• Workshops
a. Treatment Technology Alternatives
b. Local-State Nexus
c. State-Federal Roles
d. Interim Standards
e. Large-scale Considerations
• Multiple-agency document review

Along with general recommendations, this document provides specific recommendations for utilities to support their efforts to develop or improve emergency drinking water plans. The major inputs used for developing this document are listed in the accompanying text box.

4. Basic Water Supply Elements

Supplying water to the customer, under normal or emergency conditions, involves four major elements: source, treatment, storage and distribution (see Figure 1).

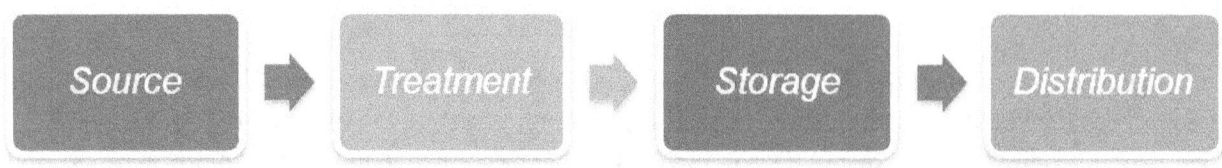

Figure 1. Basic elements for providing water.

For each element, there are specific considerations associated with procurement, implementation and operations that require evaluation (see Figure 2).

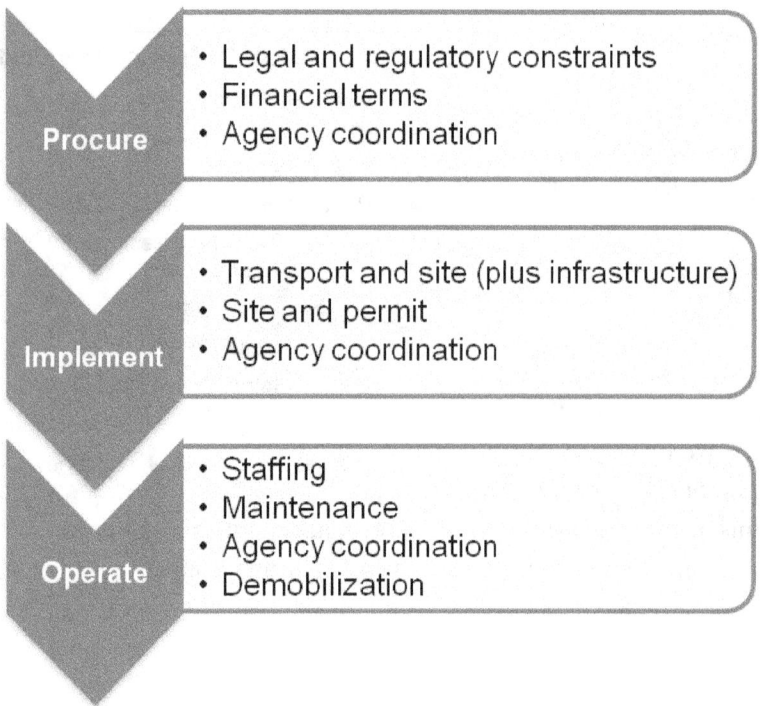

Figure 2. Considerations at each phase.

5.   Key Assumptions

Planning requires assumptions regarding:

- Water use per capita

- Time-scale of outages

- Population affected

- Water quality targets

These assumptions are discussed below.

Water Use per Capita

There are a range of values that are suggested for an emergency water supply (e.g., 0.5 gallons per person per day to 5 gallons per person per day) depending on whether water for non-drinking purposes (e.g., food preparation and hygiene) is included in the estimate. The value of 1 gallon per person per day (USACE 2006) is a plausible planning number, consistent with the Federal Emergency Management Agency (FEMA), EPA, and the Red Cross estimates for drinking, food preparation, and hygiene related to health and safety.[3] Emergency water required for fire fighting, hygiene and other needs (e.g., domestic animals), while important, is beyond the scope of this document.

> ### *Ready for a Disaster of Epic Proportions?*
>
> Large-scale disasters such as Hurricane Katrina and the 2010 earthquakes which devastated Haiti, Chile and Pakistan, and simulated disasters such as the 2008 Golden Guardian exercise in California, have demonstrated that recovery periods can be considerably greater than 21 days. For catastrophes that impact large populations, innovative solutions that have been implemented in some of the world's least developed countries[2] (WHO 2002) will have to be applied in places with developed economies as well. Such a catastrophe may require innovative approaches to scaling up mobile water treatment units, developing temporary distribution systems, or even re-location of people to areas with adequate water supply and shelter. Readying ourselves now is essential for an effective and timely response.

Time Scale of Outages

This document is intended to aid preparation for water outages lasting beyond three days, the time frame that residents would reasonably be expected to sustain themselves with their own water supply (U.S. DHS, 2009). Outages in excess of 21 days were deemed to represent a response beyond the scope of this document.

Population Considered

In certain instances, emergency water demands of urban areas may include not only the residential population, but also the day-time population of workers and tourists. The impacts and needs of critical customers (i.e. hospitals, potential shelter locations) should be considered during the planning process.

---

[2] WHO 2002. "Environmental health in emergencies and disasters: a practical guide." See discussion on p. 95.

[3] Oxfam (2010) indicates 15 L per person-day. Water, Engineering and Development Centre (Reed and Shaw 1999) suggests 3 to 5 L per person-day and FEMA (2004) indicates 1.5 gallon (5.5 L) per person-day.

Water Quality Targets

State drinking water regulations do not necessarily anticipate all possible disaster scenarios. In some instances states have found means for providing flexibility to protect the public and expedite service restoration. For short-term periods (less than 30, 60 or 90 days), an emphasis on meeting acute exposure standards only may be more appropriate than monitoring for contaminants associated with chronic, long term health risks. For planning purposes, utilities should assume that compliance with state drinking water regulations will be required unless the primacy agency issues formal regulatory relief. (See Appendix B for a summary of the workshop discussion of the applicability of SDWA drinking water standards during emergencies.)

6. Major Building Blocks for Emergency Drinking Water Plan

There are several categories of building blocks for an emergency drinking water plan, but the departure point for planning is the degree of system resilience. A critical step for planning is to identify the existing condition of system infrastructure and to reduce outage risk through system redundancy and repair capabilities.

Reducing Outage Risk through System Redundancy/Resilience and Repair Capabilities

Depending on the extent and scope of the water outage, it may be possible to compensate for partial system failures without relying on an alternate water source(s).

1. Redundant pipe connections and strategically placed valves may make it possible to isolate damaged pipes and minimize the area(s) of lost service. For example, New York City and Cleveland both rely on system redundancy for their emergency water supply plan, while Seattle has means for establishing temporary connections between pressure zones to allow by-passing of certain areas and improve the provision of service.

2. Adequate number of operable valves is essential for isolating affected parts of the system and for circumventing sources of pressure loss. Field exercises may be necessary to determine a system's valve requirements.

3. Treated water storage may also make it possible to maintain service for a certain period of time while treatment plants are repaired.

4. Emergency equipment such as generators (in the event of a power outage), fuel, or spare pipes and fittings may also make drinking water delivery via the existing water system possible. Emergency response in the aftermath of Hurricane Katrina was hampered by lack of sufficient fuel for emergency generators, and lack of ability to recharge cell phones and radios.

There are several building blocks categories that support an emergency drinking water plan: source, treatment, storage, and distribution. Each element is described separately below.

Building Blocks – Source

There are four basic source alternatives:[4]

- Local

- Neighboring Water Utilities

- Bulk Water Transport

- Pre-packaged Water

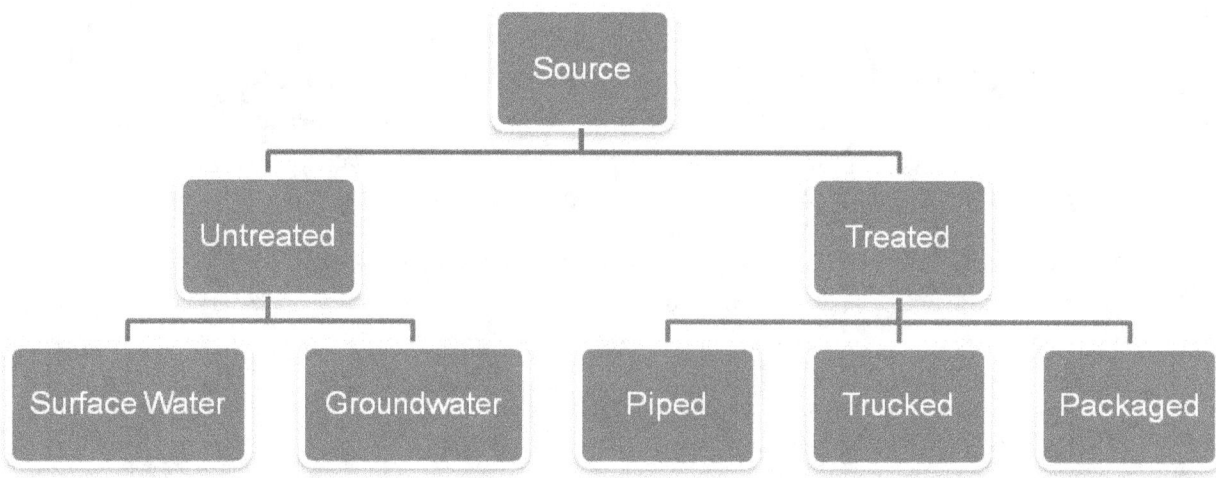

Figure 3. Source considerations.

Figure 3 illustrates another means of conceptualizing sources and starts with the question of whether they are treated or untreated.

Local Alternative Source

It may be possible to convey alternate local water sources through functioning portions of the existing water distribution system. Some cities and businesses/institutions, for example, are drilling wells for the purpose of a back-up supply in case of a water outage.[5] This type of alternative requires prior

---

[4] During outages where limited supply is available through the distribution system, it may be necessary to limit the public's water use (e.g., outdoor uses, restaurant drinking water service, bathing, cleaning clothes and dishes, flushing toilets, etc.).

[5] For example, the City of San Francisco is drilling several wells for the purpose of having connections to emergency water sources. In addition, many hospitals maintain emergency use wells on or near their facility to serve as back-up supply sources.

development of the necessary infrastructure and equipment to treat the source (if necessary), and also the means by which to connect it to the existing distribution system and transport the water. Varying system pressures and water quality parameters are also important when considering alternate sources.

Neighboring Water Utilities

Some water utilities have established interconnections with adjacent utilities. These interconnections consist of pipeline connections that allow utilities to share water resources in the event of an emergency. Examples of emergency interconnections include those between New York and New Jersey (New Jersey 2007)[6] and utilities in San Francisco Bay area.[7] In addition, some locales have devised temporary interconnections for supplying water during extreme droughts. These interconnections typically require pre-planning and written agreements between the cities/utilities that will be sharing the connection. In practice, interconnections can offer limited flexibility for larger utilities given hydraulic restrictions of the distribution network. Varying system pressures and water quality parameters are key considerations associated with the use of interconnections.

In addition, mutual aid and assistance agreements among utilities, such as a Water/Wastewater Agency Response Network (WARN), ensure that neighboring utilities can take actions to help provide an affected utility with emergency resources.[8] The purpose of a WARN is to provide a method whereby water/wastewater utilities that have sustained or anticipate damages from natural or human-caused incidents can provide and receive emergency aid and assistance in the form of personnel, equipment, materials, and other associated services as necessary from other water/wastewater utilities.

Bulk Water

Bulk water focuses on transporting treated water, though untreated water could conceivably be transported as well. Treated water can be from existing treated water reservoirs, treatment plants, or nearby utilities. Options for bulk water transport include water bladders, tankers/milk trucks, and water buffaloes. For potable water, tanks should meet NSF/ANSI Standard 61 (NSF International/American National Standards Institute). Licensed bulk water haulers or food grade tank haulers may offer the best option in emergencies. Milk or potable water tanker trucks are preferred, but trucks designed for transport of other food products are also acceptable. Sanitation requirements for these trucks are state-specific, and most states have their own water hauling guidelines (e.g., Oregon, Connecticut, and Missouri all have web-accessible guidelines). The requirements of the state in which the plan is being developed should be consulted. The Centers for Disease Control and Prevention (CDC) makes reference to both the World Health Organization's "Cleaning and disinfecting water storage tanks and tankers"[9]

---

[6] NJDEP. 2007. Interconnection Study Mitigation of Water Supply Emergencies – Public Version.

[7] East Bay Municipal Utility District. Inter-Agency Intertie Projects. http://www.ebmud.com/about-ebmud/news/project-updates/inter-agency-intertie-projects (Accessed January 14, 2011.)

[8] Mutual aid and assistance agreements exist in 47 states and the National Capitol Region see www.NationalWARN.org (Accessed February 14, 2011.)

[9] WHO. 2005. "Cleaning and disinfecting water storage tanks and tankers". Technical Notes for Emergencies, Technical Note No. 3. Revised July 1, 2005. Accessed May 10, 2010. Avalable: http://www.searo.who.int/LinkFiles/List_of_Guidelines_for_Health_Emergency_Cleaning_and_disinfecting_water_storage_tanks.pdf

(WHO 2005) and Connecticut's "Bulk Water Hauling Guidelines" (Connecticut 2008).[10] In the aftermath of Hurricane Katrina, many dirty potable water tanker trucks were sent to the Gulf Region due to confusion over where and when truck cleaning was expected to take place. Developing contractual agreements with water haulers in advance should be part of emergency preparation.

Pre-packaged Water

Bottled water sources can be stored on-hand, transported into the affected area in the event of an emergency, or a combination of the two. Many states maintain a list of approved vendors.[11] Arrangements for transportation from off-site should be made in advance via contract; this can help prevent "double counting," such that multiple agencies are not relying on the same water in the event of a large-scale emergency. There are a range of possible sizes for packaged water. Selection of size will depend on a number of factors including handling, availability, and cost. [12] Since a pre-packaged water strategy can be implemented quickly, it has often been the preferred strategy. In the case of more extended outages, however, such a strategy may not be sustainable. Nevertheless, it can be the first phase of the response until temporary repairs, modifications, or other water supply options can be implemented.

Summary

The different water supply building blocks will be paired with distribution methods, depending on the condition of the existing infrastructure. Table 1 summarizes these alternatives.

Table 1. Alternate Water Supply Characterization

Water Source	Distribution Method	
	Through Existing System	*Special Sites*
Normal Source	• System redundancy/resilience • Emergency equipment (e.g., generators, replacement piping) • Extra storage • Household treatment (e.g., bleach, iodine tablets, boiling, point-of-use device)	Treated water obtained from hydrants or reservoirs and transported to un-serviceable areas
Local Alternate Source	Emergency/pre-existing connections to distribution system (with or without additional treatment) for groundwater or surface water	With or without additional treatment for groundwater or surface water
Neighboring Utility (Including Bulk Water)	Pipe interconnection with neighboring water utility	Mutual aid agreement – treated water transported to designated sites
Pre-packaged Water	Not applicable	Vendor contracts or federal assistance

---

[10] Connecticut Department of Public Health Drinking Water Section. 2008. "Bulk Water Hauling Guidelines." Effective February 1, 2008. Accessed May 10, 2010. http://www.ct.gov/dph/lib/dph/drinking_water/pdf/Bulk_Water_Hauling_Guidelines.pdf .

[11] For example, the California Department of Public Health, Food and Drug Branch maintain a list of approved water haulers and vendors.

[12] For example, California Office of Emergency Services recommends that packages of 1gallon be used, if possible, while Seattle uses 1.5 gallon bags in their emergency drinking water system.

Basic Building Blocks – Treatment

The treatment considerations are organized under two categories: (1) centralized or satellite (i.e., distributed) treatment and (2) point-of-use treatment (see Figure 4). The regulatory determination as to whether a source is approved by regulatory authorities for potable use is critical. Discussion of considerations for each building block is presented below.

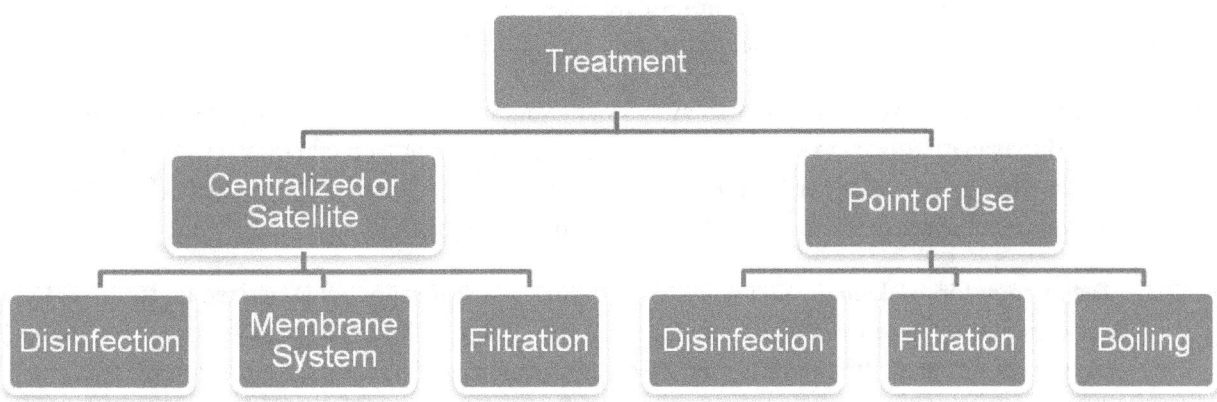

Figure 4. Treatment considerations.

Centralized or Satellite Treatment Options

Large-scale treatment options include low pressure membrane filtration (i.e., microfiltration and ultrafiltration) and high pressure membranes (e.g., reverse osmosis). For example, the Department of Defense (DOD) and some state National Guard units maintain water purification systems that are typically used to for troop support during overseas troop deployment, but the systems can sometimes be deployed in a domestic emergency. In addition, the private sector has a wide-range of products and has experience deploying under various disaster scenarios. Utilities and others should take into consideration the various procedural requirements to prepare the treatment units for deployment, such as the example provided in California's "Multi-Agency Response Guidance for Emergency Drinking Water Procurement & Distribution" (California 2007).[13] The scale and duration of an event and the associated recovery phase are important parameters in determining an appropriate drinking water strategy. Depending on the risks, a utility may consider various alternative strategies that address the plausible ranges of outages.

Discussion with vendors and procurement specialists during the workshops indicated that if packaged treatment systems are not pre-purchased or planned, procurement in response to an emergency event could be delayed due to unfamiliarity with the equipment. Many manufacturers maintain pilot treatment

---

[13] California Office of Emergency Services. 2007. "Multi-Agency Response Guidance for Emergency Drinking Water Procurement & Distribution" Accessed January 14, 2011
http://www.oes.ca.gov/Operational/OESHome.nsf/PDF/Drinking%20Water%20Guidance/$file/DrinkWaterGd.pdf

units that could be dispatched in an emergency, but depending on desired capacity and requirements, deployment and refurbishment typically takes several weeks. Purchase of units designed for the treatment requirements of a specific raw water source can require up to three months for delivery. It is essential to determine whether ancillary items (i.e., pumps, piping and fittings, and chlorine disinfection) are included with packaged treatment units. Some vendors provide self-contained, integrated treatment units that can become fully-functional upon arrival. However, the affected utility will typically play a central role in making the connection between the treatment system unit and their existing infrastructure.

There are critical constraints on the rapid, large-scale response for providing a drinking water supply during an emergency. Planners should address these constraints head-on:

1. Assuming that the water distribution system will not be intact, the emergency response default for drinking water has been to provide bottled water. However, at a certain disaster scale, duration, or remediation-recovery period, this strategy becomes unsustainable. The trigger(s) for different response strategies should be considered before disaster strikes.

2. Technology for producing water on-site is available in the form of containerized units, typically consisting of hybrid membrane systems (i.e., low pressure followed by high pressure membrane units, or micro/ultrafiltration followed by reverse osmosis). The initial purification process can also be followed by granulated activated carbon or ultraviolet treatment (or limestone contactor for pH stabilization), then chlorination.

3. Sources of treatment units may include the military (U.S. Army), State National Guard, and/or private sector vendors. The U.S. Army has capacity to support its current soldier strength. It is very difficult to predict military equipment availability for local emergencies.

4. Any treatment system should be coupled with means of storage, packaging, and distribution. Efforts at packaging in the field include molding plastic bottles as an integral part of packaging (the U.S. Army is evaluating several alternatives). The logistics of distributing water to the affected population may pose significant challenges.

5. Additional things that should be addressed include:

    a. Treatment unit performance certification

    b. State acceptance of sources, treatment packages, and operations (Raw water quality is a key factor influencing the approval of a source-treatment combination.)

    c. Procurement mechanisms and execution

    d. Identification and preparation of treatment sites with all ancillary facilities for water abstraction, power, plumbing, residuals management and security

    e. Strategy for water distribution

Recommendations to address these items are found in Section 9.

Point-of-Use Treatment

In some cases, home treatment of drinking water may be sufficient in an emergency situation. For example, if both electrical power and piped water are available, boil water notices may be appropriate, and emergency water distribution may not be needed. Other home treatment options exist, such as hypochlorite (i.e., bleach) treatment, distribution of iodine tablets to individuals or use of manual filtration devices (e.g., backpacker filters, Lifestraw® [Vestergaard Frandsen Inc.]). However, point-of-use (POU) devices are not currently accepted by most state regulatory agencies for treatment compliance. In any case, it is possible that point-of-use treatment will be used by individuals in addition to the emergency water supply provided. If POU devices are used by individual consumers, they should be cautioned to obtain devices certified under NSF International Standard 53.

Basic Building Blocks – Storage

Some form of storage is necessary, whether it is downstream of treatment units prior to distribution or for bulk water (see Figure 5). For packaged water, there may be a need for warehousing the water prior to moving it to distribution sites. In some cases, water from existing treated water reservoirs can be pumped into tankers or packaged on-site to meet customer needs. Forklifts and other equipment will be required to transfer the water into tankers or loading pallets onto trucks.

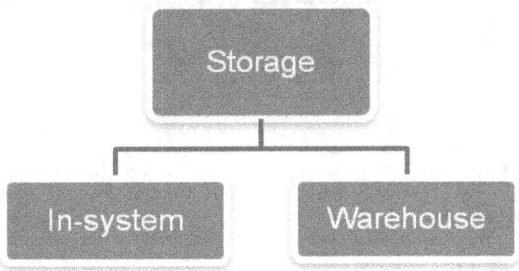

Figure 5. Storage considerations.

Basic Building Blocks – Distribution

A critical step for identifying which water distribution options are appropriate is to determine the post-disaster condition of the local infrastructure.

▶ *On-line* – One set of water distribution options requires the use of all or part of the existing water distribution system. This depends on the configuration of the existing water distribution system in the affected area, the accessibility of alternative pipelines for moving the water, and the availability of valve control options for isolating affected areas and re-routing water.

▶ *Off-line* – The other set of water distribution options is triggered when the water distribution system is damaged to the point where it is not practical to use it for distribution. This requires importing water for distribution at local sites. This type of "off-line" distribution requires the coordination of water transport and water distribution sites.

A summary of all available water distribution options, for on-line or off-line scenarios, is depicted in Figure 6. The on-line/off-line distinction is critical to option evaluation and emergency assessment. However, Figure 6 shows that water from various sources could be distributed either through an existing, partially- operating distribution system, or via distribution sites.

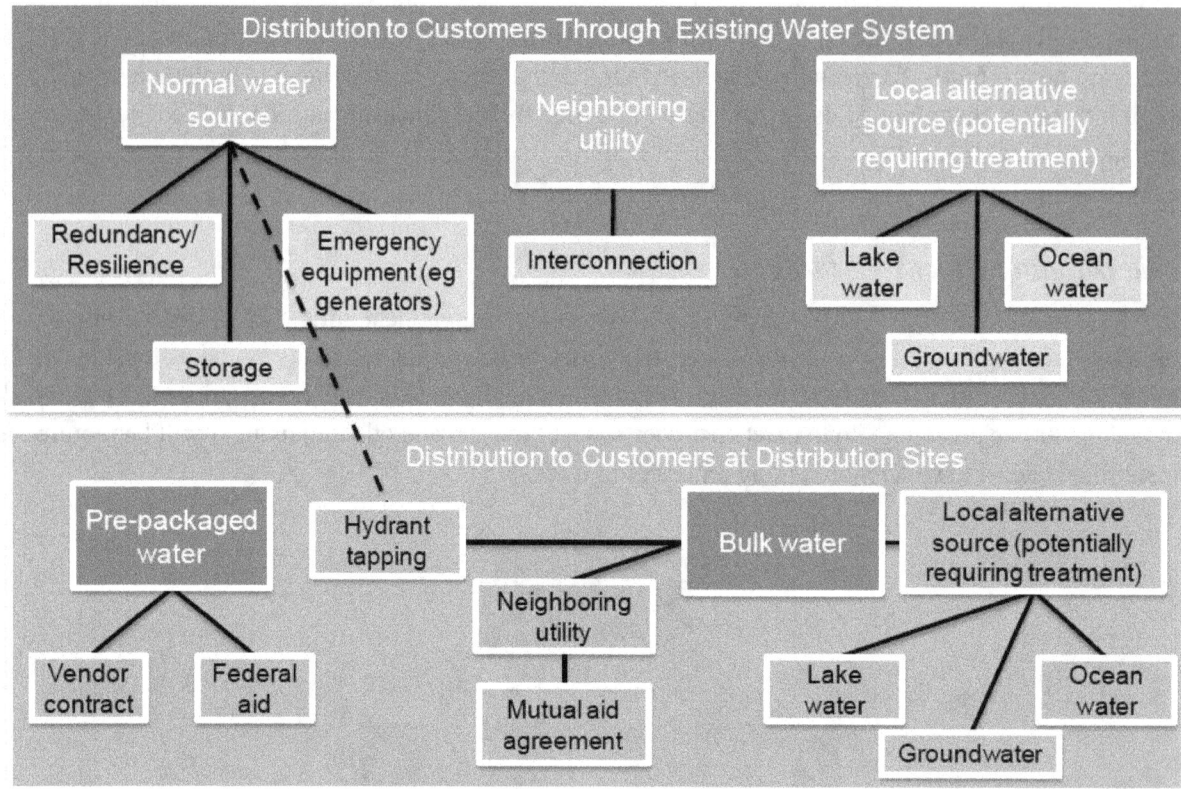

Figure 6. Water distribution options.

Depending on the nature of the damage and the ability of a utility to make functioning pipe connections, it may be impossible to transport water from functioning to non-functioning portions of the distribution system. If uncontaminated water is in sufficient supply within the existing water system, but cannot be distributed as needed, the water may need to be tapped at fire hydrants or other locations within the functioning system for local distribution, and/or moved in bulk water tankers.

There are a variety of logistical considerations for off-line distribution (see Figure 7). These are discussed below. Other emergency response programs may also already have plans in place for distribution of other emergency supplies. Therefore, for off-line water distribution, it may be beneficial to coordinate with other local emergency response programs.

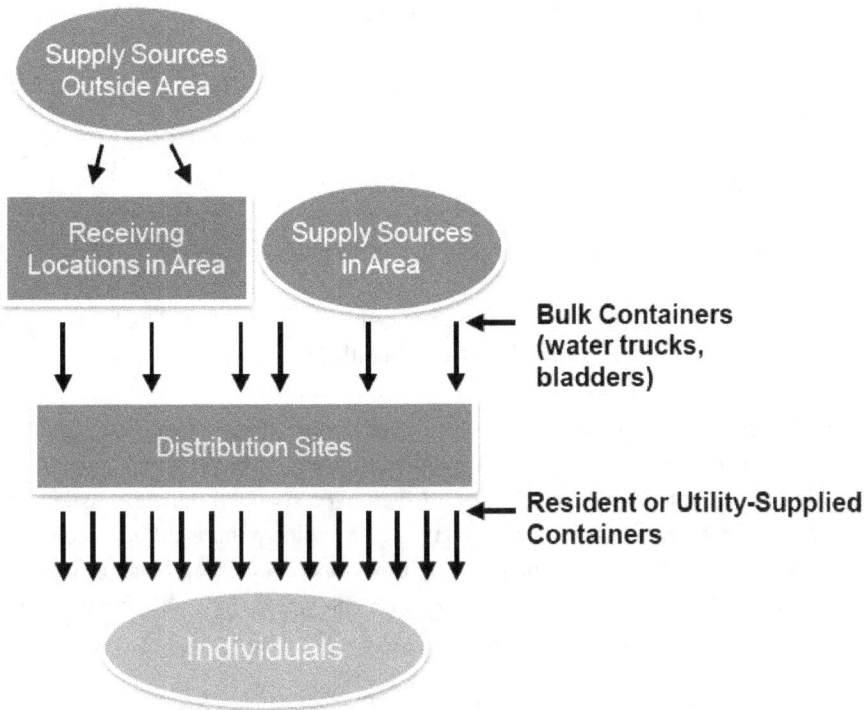

Figure 7. Overview of transportation and distribution flow.

Packaging

Bulk potable water sources can be packaged for individual use before distribution (either at their sources or at staging areas), or they can be distributed in bulk directly from large containers to individual customer's containers via spigots. Bottling or bagging facilities can also be used to expedite distribution of pre-packaged water. Issues that could limit the practicality and effectiveness of on-site water bottling include availability of containers, material selection and certification, operator certification from the state primacy agency, and testing-monitoring requirements.

Seattle's Emergency Drinking Water Distribution Planning

As part of their emergency planning, the Seattle Public Utilities (SPU) has developed a three-fold strategy for supplying water in an emergency:

1. Interconnections with neighboring water utilities

2. On hand supplies of NSF-certified portable flexible piping to bridge/bypass breaks

3. Emergency water provisioning either using trucked 3,500 gallon bladders for filling customer's containers or using contracts to obtain pallets of bottled water for distribution

This last option involves using customized packaging equipment to fill disposable plastic bags at key locations throughout the city. In an event impacting more than 1000 households, citizens would come to the location to pick up their water in SPU-supplied, vacuum sealed, FDA-approved six-quart puncture sealed bags. The maximum number of people that can be served at any given distribution point is 20,000 people per day (assuming 650 vehicles). The staffing requirements for a distribution point are not insignificant (e.g., over 70 people for a 24 hour shift). SPU has six systems available for deployment. SPU has conducted numerous exercises to better coordinate and streamline responses.

Source: Pat O'Brien, Seattle Public Utilities (May 11, 2010)

Site Identification and Set-up

Proper planning of emergency water distribution sites is essential. After Hurricane Katrina, bottled water was plentiful, but did not reach the public efficiently due to poorly planned distribution.

Some features ideal for distribution sites include: open space, emergency shelters and schools, locations near fire hydrants, easy road access, and good lighting. Fire stations, police stations, and other government agencies undertaking emergency response activities are not recommended as distribution sites. Some have suggested that property controlled by the local government and property near commercial water suppliers should not be selected. Placing distribution sites near commercial water suppliers (e.g., grocery stores) might create redundancy. A number of criteria should be considered for site selection. For example, the California Office of Emergency Services, referring to the Los Angeles County Fire Department's "Sample Local Drinking Water Distribution Plan,"[14] (California 2007) included the following considerations:

*   200 x 200 foot minimum area
*   Paved surface
*   Accessible by truck
*   Access restricted by curbs
*   Electricity and phone service, if possible

---

[14] California (2007), the Governor's Office of Emergency Services referring to the Los Angeles County Fire Department's "Sample Local Drinking Water Distribution Plan."

- Ease of transportation to and from

- Accessible to tractor-trailer rigs

- Central and accessible to the community

- Geographic distribution of sites proportionate to population density

- Close to elderly and critical care facilities

The 200 x 200 foot minimum area is consistent with the U.S. Army Corps of Engineers (USACE) recommended space requirement for a single loading point. USACE recommends staging multiple loading points together, increasing the size of individual distribution sites. A sample distribution site is shown in Figure 8.

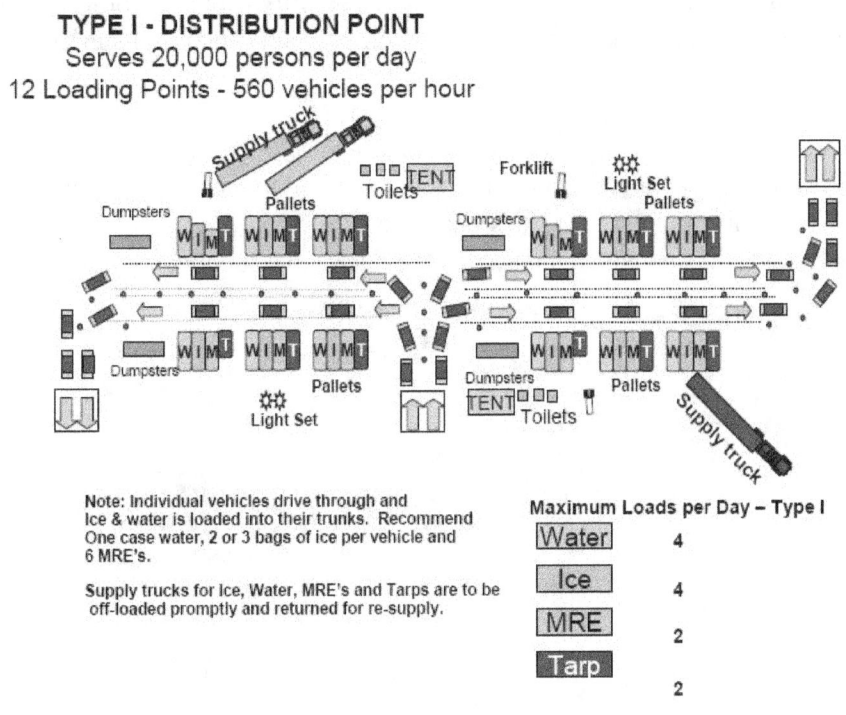

Source: "Emergency Support Function (ESF) #3 Field Guide." Page 68 (USACE, 2006)

Figure 8. Example point of distribution.

Equipment

The equipment needed for emergency water distribution includes at a minimum, the following: portable radios (with batteries and chargers), tactical radio frequencies, cellular phones (with batteries and chargers), flat-bed trailers with tractors and drivers, forklifts with operators, fuel, word processing computers, fax machine, phone line, photo-copy machine, and a communications trailer (California

2007).[15] The recommended equipment listed in the "ESF #3 Field Guide" (USACE 2006) includes pallet jacks, power light sets, toilets, tents, dumpsters, traffic cones, and two-way radios.

Staffing

Adequate staffing is essential. Roles and responsibilities are varied and some positions require equipment operator expertise. However, it may be possible to augment the staff at distribution sites using utility customer service personnel, neighborhood emergency response team volunteers, or aid from outside agencies such as the Red Cross. Additional suggestions can be found in "Water Security Initiative: Interim Guidance on Developing Consequence Management Plans for Drinking Water Utilities" (EPA 2008).

Security

A security force may be needed both for protecting water supplies and controlling crowds at distribution sites. Local law enforcement should be consulted regarding their ability to perform this duty during an emergency, but others might be needed. A contract with a local security firm for contract guard services could be considered as a contingency in planning for protection of emergency water supplies.

Summary

Determining the condition of the existing distribution system is important in developing an appropriate distribution strategy. For planning purposes, utilities should to consider situations where the distribution system is partially useable or even completely unusable. The alternative supply options are summarized in Table 2.

---

[15] California (2007).
http://www.oes.ca.gov/Operational/OESHome.nsf/PDF/Drinking%20Water%20Guidance/$file/DrinkWaterGd.pdf

Table 2. Alternative Water Supply Options

Option*	Description	Implementation Requirements	Capacity/Scalability
Bottled Water	Distribute bottled water at distribution sites.	Vendor contract or contract agreement with other utilities for aid	Determined by vendor availability and local storage capacity (if storing bottles on-site)
Reverse osmosis	Treat saline water sources, such as saline ground water and ocean water.	• Water source • Power source • Mode of transport to distribution sites	0.5-1.0 MGD units
Filtration	Treat untreated local water sources by ultrafiltration, microfiltration, GAC, or other filtration methods.	• Water source • Pumps/intake • Chemicals • Power source • Operators • Distribution points (into system or to packaging)	0.5-1.0 MGD
Point-of-Use Treatment	Use boil water notices for contamination that can be treated by boiling. Other options include household bleach disinfection, purification tablets or manual filters.	• Power in customer homes • Functioning distribution system	Applicable over any scale demand
Bottle In-house	Bulk water can be bottled at the source prior to transport and/or distribution.	• Bulk supply of water • Power source • Packaging material • Operators	Up to 120 packages per minute (2.5 gal or less) (300 gpm ~ 0.4 mgd)
Bag In-house	Bulk water can be bagged at the source prior to transport and/or distribution.	• Bulk supply of water • Power source • Two operators	1-2.5 gal bags, 12-15 bags/min
Stationary bladders	Distribution can take place at the water source from large (not transportable) bladders.	• Water source near an appropriate distribution site • Pipe and spigot apparatus • Individuals must bring containers • Staffing and operators	10,000-100,000 gal
Bladder transport to distribution sites	Small bladders that can be transported on a truck bed can be brought to distribution sites.	• Local water source • Pipe and spigot apparatus • Individuals must bring containers • Truck beds appropriate for transporting full bladders and forklifts, etc. • Functioning roadways	Up to 6,000 gal
Transport in tanker-trucks	Utilities can make agreements with companies in the area that have access to potable tanker trucks (e.g., dairy trucks) – or may have some on hand.	• Contract with company to use trucks in an emergency • Potable water source • Distribution method (e.g., packaging on-site) • Functioning roadways	3,000-20,000 gal

* Costs will depend on multiple factors including size, duration, site conditions, equipment availability, security considerations, and degree of infrastructure required.

7.   Process for Developing Utility-Specific Plans

The process for developing an EDWP entails narrowing the options and identifying the most appropriate elements of the utility's "portfolio" of assets and the steps required to use those assets in an emergency. In addition, there are several steps that precede the actual formulation of the strategy for a utility-specific EDWP. These steps include:

1. ***Determine the Potential Need***: What is maximum plausible extent of outages based on the risks for a given location? Does this assessment consider the potential that future events may be more severe than the historical record indicates (e.g., notion of what constitutes a 500-year storm may be changing). What levels of service can realistically be provided following the event? How long will it take for restoration efforts to meet the targeted levels of service?

    The vulnerability assessment conducted by a utility will inform the magnitude and duration of the events being considered, and, therefore, the alternatives that will be most relevant. The ANSI/ASME-ITI/AWWA J100-10 Risk Analysis and Management for Critical Asset Protection (RAMCAP®) Standard for Risk and Resilience Management of Water and Wastewater Systems should be consulted. Some of the natural hazards cited in J100 include earthquakes, floods, hurricanes, tornadoes, wildfires, ice storms, and others that affect specific locations (e.g., mudslides). Some of the malevolent threats cited in J100 include terrorism, crime and serious vandalism.

2. ***Assess the Gap***: Based on the existing population and the targeted level of service post-disaster, along with the targeted quantities and quality of water, what gap in resources will exist for a potable water supply? (One effective method for identifying these gaps is to conduct table-top emergency preparedness exercises.)

3. ***Communicate the Gap***: Has that gap been communicated to local and state emergency management and other stakeholders? Having all stakeholders understand the evaluation of event scenarios and gaps facing a water utility is critical for building partnerships that will facilitate the planning and implementation phases of the emergency water supply strategies.

4. ***Identify a Water Supply Strategy to Bridge the Gap***: Using the approach shown in Figure 9, a portfolio of options can be formulated and considered for implementation. This process requires that the following questions be addressed: What specific resources will be needed to bridge the water supply gap, and what alternatives make most sense? Based on the building blocks for an emergency drinking water plan detailed in Section 6 (source, treatment, storage, distribution) along with the assessment of magnitude and duration of outages, an options portfolio is developed. There is a need to identify particular constraints limiting the applicability of the Section 6 building blocks. After screening out building blocks, further refinement of options can be based on utility-specific evaluation criteria and possibly weighting factors for evaluating the alternatives. For example, Figure 10 provides rating criteria that can be applied to each option to make a comparative assessment of all possible alternatives. The outcome may not be a single supply option, but an array of options bundled into a portfolio. A portfolio strategy accounts for differences in scale and duration of the potential responses.

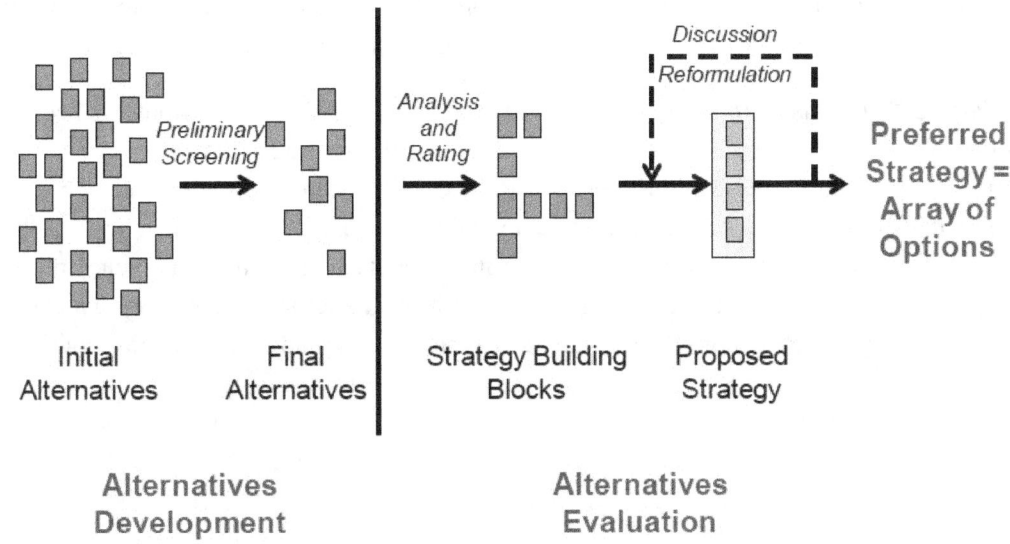

Figure 9. Identifying most appropriate strategy.

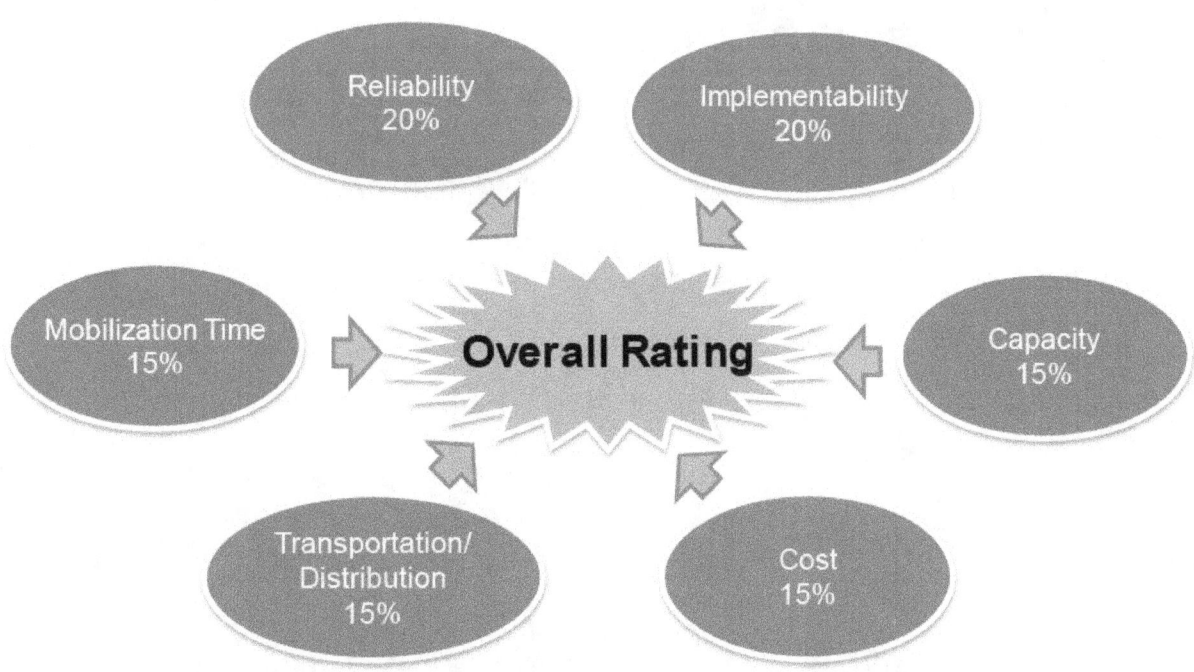

Figure 10. Example evaluation criteria and weighing factors.

5. ***Prepare to Implement the Water Supply Strategy:*** The plan should address how external resources will be managed (e.g., receiving, locating and staffing) and how the utility will coordinate with local emergency units on points of distribution (PODs). Addressing siteing, ancillary requirements (e.g., power, security, storage), and regulatory pre-approvals up front is essential for being able to requisition and assimilate external assistance during an emergency.

6. ***Prioritize Initial Local Investments:*** Once a portfolio of water supply options has been identified for a utility, the final step in developing an EDWP is prioritizing any advance actions/investments that can speed the response in the event of a disaster. This step involves evaluating the risk of an event, the likelihood that such an investment would prove useful, the costs, and whether there are other benefits for advance actions/preparation/investments additional to emergency preparedness (e.g., an interconnect or intertie may provide benefit as an alternate supply during a capital project or serve as a temporary supply during routine distribution system maintenance activities).

8.   Capabilities during a Crisis

Identifying the capabilities of the various actors is essential to both developing an EDWP and identifying appropriate levels of emergency preparedness. Equally essential is identifying all potential resources available along with the procedures for accessing those resources. In the event of an emergency, local authorities can be overwhelmed and may need outside assistance. The response should be tailored to the severity of the event and projected duration of the recovery phase. As such, planning might involve multiple agencies – including local, state, and federal agencies – as well as NGOs. The primary mission of the utility is to restore piped water service. They will likely be dependent on others to provide and distribute emergency water supplies. However, the utility will still likely retain some responsibility in the planning capacity and as liaison between their customer base and the operations supplying the emergency water.

The Local Utility

In the process of developing an EDWP as a part of their overall emergency response plan, the utility should communicate with all relevant government agencies, NGOs, and stakeholders. The utility should also take the lead in assuring the procurement of aid agreements and necessary supply and service contracts. Within the EDWP, a local Emergency Operations Center (EOC) should be identified. The EOC is the point of contact for coordination with all external aid during an emergency.

One of the primary goals of utilities in the aftermath of an emergency should be to restore piped water service. A good EDWP should avoid resource allocation conflicts (i.e., personnel and equipment) during a disaster in order to allow the utility to focus on restoring piped water service expeditiously.

State Agencies

Given that each state has its own procedures and regulations, the utilities should communicate with all applicable state agencies in the process of developing their emergency response plan. EPA's Water Security Initiative (EPA 2008) lists the agencies with a role, or a potential role, in emergency response plans and in the provision of emergency water supplies in Table D-2 (re-printed below as Table 3).

Table 3. State Agency Roles and Responsibilities

Partner Organizations	*Roles and Responsibilities*
Drinking water and wastewater primacy agencies	Primacy agencies can be public health agencies as well as separate State or local environmental agencies, such as State or regional water quality boards. [In a] contamination [scenario], there may be regulatory ramifications related to use of contaminated water, public notification, environmental concerns for discharged water, quality of alternative supplies, and other issues. Additionally, the primacy agency, along with EPA, should be consulted on any potential remediation and recovery plan.
Environmental and public health laboratories	Provide analytical support during consequence management including credibility determination, response and remediation. State public health laboratories provide access to CDC's Laboratory Response Network.
State government	May have a role in establishing formal agreements with state partners or coordinating funding resources. Should be informed and engaged once contamination has been confirmed to assist in coordination of resources and communication.
State emergency responders	Provide support if a contamination incident is confirmed. Should be engaged in consequence management planning to ensure efficient transition in the event that a contamination incident escalates. State Emergency Response Commissions (SERCs) can be identified by contacting Emergency Planning and Community Right-to-Know Act (EPCRA) hotline at 800-535-0202. LEPCs report up to the SERCs.
State emergency management and homeland security agencies	Provide support if a contamination incident is confirmed. Should be engaged in consequence management planning to ensure efficient transition in the event that a contamination incident escalates.
State law enforcement	Provide support if a contamination incident is confirmed. Should be engaged in consequence management planning to ensure efficient transition in the event that a contamination incident escalates.
State Department of Health	Can track data used to determine if there is a public health incident? Can alert health care providers of potential contamination incidents and appropriate treatment methods.
State environmental representative	Could be located in the public health department or the engineering department. Can provide guidance on engineering devices which could be used in cleanup as well as monitoring wells/devices which can be used to determine the extent of contamination.
Local National Guard units	Can provide assistance in cordoning off quarantined or contaminated areas and may be key to alternate water supply acquisition and distribution.

Source: U.S. EPA. (2008). Water Security Initiative: Interim Guidance on Developing Consequence Management Plans for Drinking Water Utilities. Page 86.Federal Response: Emergency Support Functions

Under provisions of the Stafford Act, a state governor can request federal assistance. FEMA will coordinate activities with other federal agencies as depicted in Figure 11. The relevant activities might include:

1. Providing technical assistance

2. Participating in a multi-agency coordination

3. Coordinating water staging/distribution sites

4. Delivering water to staging areas/distribution sites, the distribution process

5. Procuring water purification equipment, supplies and other materials

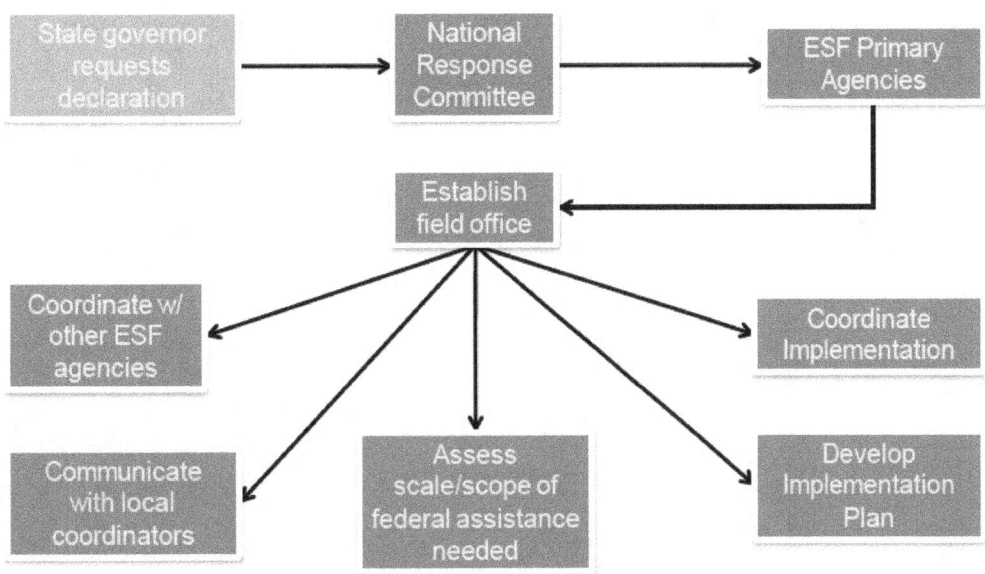

Figure 11. Roles and responsibilities in the National Response Framework.

Federal Agencies

Emergency response actions under the National Response Framework (NRF) (see Figure 11) are divided into several different Emergency Support Functions (ESFs). There are a total of 15 different ESFs, each with their own lead federal agency and scope of work. The two ESFs that apply directly to emergency water supplies are ESF #3: Public Works and Engineering, and ESF #8: Health and Medical Services. Each NRF Annex includes a detailed description of ESF duties, procedures, and organizations, which are available on FEMA's website (FEMA 2008; FEMA 2003).[16] After a federal declaration of emergency, a joint field office (JFO) is established. The JFO determines the scale of the federal assistance needed to meet official state requests and coordinates the response. The lead agency of ESF #3 is the U.S. Army Corps of Engineers. The Corps coordinates its efforts with other federal agencies, including EPA and the U.S. Public Health Service (FEMA, 2008). Services and supplies provided might include emergency generators, bottled or bulk water, ice, and emergency large-scale water treatment facilities (USACE, 2006). The lead agency for ESF #8 (Public Health) is the U.S. Department of Health and Human Services (U.S. Public Health Service) through the Assistant Secretary for Public Health Emergency Preparedness (ASPHER).

Under the Stafford Act, emergency response activities are typically financed 90% by the federal government and 10% by local government. Long-term infrastructure restoration is typically financed at 75% by the federal government and 25% by the local government.

Other Aid Agencies

---

[16] FEMA National Response Framework Resource Center. http://www.fema.gov/emergency/nrf/

The Red Cross, the Salvation Army, and other community service NGOs often assist federal emergency responders, and they should be included as stakeholders in developing the EDWP.

9. Key Workshop Findings

During the development of this document, a series of workshops were held with water utilities; first responders; equipment manufacturers; and officials from local, regional, state and federal government agencies to elicit observations concerning the provision of emergency water supplies following a major disaster. The discussion participants identified eight key findings that can assist in expediting the provision of emergency water supplies. These key findings are displayed in Table 4.

Table 4. Summary of Key Findings

	Description
I	Assess the potential impacts of each disaster scenario on the population served.
II	Utilities, in close coordination with local and state agencies, should develop plans to assure reasonable provision of emergency water supplies.
III	Local agencies should integrate loss of water service into their planning exercises.
IV	Better information is needed on the scope and magnitude of forecasted disasters and risk scenarios on potable water needs.
V	Identify the gap between projected needs, local capacity, and available state-federal and NGO resources to better plan for post-disaster emergency water supply.
VI	Aggregate gaps identified at local and state levels to assess existing and supplemental resources for emergency water supply.
VII	Highlight the need for personal preparedness of citizens, including the need for a 3-to-5 day supply of potable water.
VIII	Develop strategies for improving the efficiency of providing emergency potable water.

Finding I - Assess the potential impacts of each disaster scenario on the population served by each water utility.

Determine the Potential for Extended Outages – The risk assessment[17] should include reasonable worst-case events, whether they be hurricanes, floods, fires, earthquakes or terrorism, in terms of the severity of damage, the impacted populations, and the anticipated duration until full service is restored. This assessment should make it possible to (a) identify local preparation and mitigation actions and (b) understand the point at which local resources are exhausted and external assistance is required.

Communicate the Anticipated Need to Other Agencies – After an assessment of the risks and local capacities to respond, utilities should communicate the magnitude and duration of potable water requirements to local, state, and federal agencies and identify the point at which external resources will be necessary.

---

[17] ANSI/ASME-ITI/AWWA J100-10 Risk Analysis and Management for Critical Asset Protection (RAMCAP®) Standard for Risk and Resilience Management of Water and Wastewater Systems.

Finding II –   Utilities, in close coordination with local and state authorities, should make reasonable provision of an emergency water supply.

Following this document, a utility should develop a plan that addresses which potable water alternatives (i.e., encompassing sources, treatment, and distribution) are the most feasible for the maximum credible events, how these alternatives would be implemented, and the roles-responsibilities of its staff versus external staff (i.e., regional, state, federal agencies, or NGOs). Some of items that should be considered in an emergency drinking water plan include:

- Coordination of procurement of emergency water supplies;
- Distribution locations (PODs, bulk water delivery points, storage);
- Determining where water can be injected hydraulically into system; and
- Identifying potential locations for containerized units and for providing necessary grading, power, and security.

The emergency drinking water plan should be created in coordination with and in awareness of regional and state emergency response officials.

Finding III –   Integrate loss of water service into local planning exercises.

Planning exercises should be specific to relative to water needs. Agencies should identify and accommodate the necessary equipment, approvals, and personnel required to respond to the scenario. This includes but is not limited to:

- Assessing potential locations for distributing water with respect to scenarios only involving water and scenarios involving full-scale responses (e.g., temporary housing);
- Procuring equipment (e.g., generators, containerized treatment, or packaging units);
- Addressing coordination with other agencies and issues such as transportation, staffing, crowd control and security; and
- Developing communication protocols for describing situations, locations for obtaining water, water quality, etc.

Finding IV –   Need for better information regarding the scope and magnitude of forecasted disasters impacting potable water.

Understand the Potential for Extended Outages – As water utilities and cities assess their own vulnerabilities and forecasted recovery periods, they need to confirm their expectations for assistance from others, given the logistical complexity involved in providing drinking water.

To that end, it would be beneficial to promote state-wide and regional exercises that specifically consider water outages. A few opportunities include:

- *The National Level Exercise (NLE) 2011* – This exercise provides an opportunity to incorporate water system failures so as to: (a) examine various interdependencies associated with a response and (b) critically examine availability of key equipment that may have limited availability or long lead time for procurement (e.g., microturbines, pumps, generators).
- *FEMA Regional Interagency Steering Committee (RISC) Meetings* – Serving to coordinate interagency and intergovernmental issues related to disaster planning and operations, meetings

focused on water outages would afford opportunities to better sensitize state-federal agencies to the scope and need.

- *State Emergency Response Plan (ERP) Review* – EPA and FEMA should coordinate review and evaluation of ERPs with state drinking water and emergency management officials.
- *Water/Wastewater Agency Response Network (WARNs)* – States can better coordinate with WARNs to identify needs/gaps involving primacy agencies, state emergency management agencies, and other critical agencies. WARNs should be involved in state and regional exercise planning, implementation, and after-action reporting. Creating incentives for WARNs to provide training and conduct exercises for the broad spectrum of utilities within their state would also be beneficial.
- *National Incident Management System (NIMS)* - Provide additional training on a state and association level to reinforce integration of NIMS structure into emergency response program. Incentivize utilities and WARNS through state and federal grants.

Assess the Significance of Extended Outages – Multi-agency emergency water supply plans should include an assessment as to recovery periods being extended due to critical spare parts not being available for long durations and the time periods for restoring critical infrastructure to functional condition. Consequently, provision of potable water and other measures will be required for greater durations than those conventionally planned.

State and federal agencies should coordinate a formal study assessing the impacts of extended outages on economic and public health. This will include three steps. First, the local costs of extended loss of water service should be calculated including industry, businesses, and the utility. Second, impacts on public health should be assessed starting with local vulnerability assessments. Third, the costs/damages should be compared to the costs of mitigating the impacts. These efforts would build on findings from California's Golden Guardian exercise in November 2008 and the USACE/FEMA Senior Leadership Seminar in April 2010.

Finding V - Need to develop understanding of the gaps between projected needs, local capacity and state-federal and NGO resources in order to adequately plan for post-disaster provision of potable water.

As cities and utilities assess their infrastructure vulnerabilities and the consequences of plausible disaster scenarios, states should aggregate the projected assistance needs that could be requested. The gap between local resources and the projected need requires careful, joint evaluation by state primacy and emergency management agencies. The evaluation should identify triggers to manage resource needs in coordination with local emergency management agencies. The regional offices of EPA and FEMA should be incorporated so that functional relationships are established and a shared understanding of impact potential is communicated.

A starting point for identifying state response capacity may be for the state drinking water administrator to present water utility risk analyses to state emergency management and National Guard units and discuss with them the resourcing strategy.

Finding VI –   Based on gaps identified at local levels and aggregated at state levels, there is a need to assess existing and supplemental resources for water provisioning.

Resources necessary to provide post-disaster potable water are available in various public and private forms. State and federal agencies should, in a coordinated manner, assess the capacity of federal, state, and local resources for addressing the potential needs. This might include evaluating military resources and National Guard resources and mobilization times. It should also include private sector/vendor capacity as either a supplementary element of the strategy or as part of a contingency plan.[18]

Finding VII - Highlight the need for personal preparedness of citizens, including the need for a three-to-five day supply of potable water.

While it is well understood in emergency management field that there will be time lag between the need for potable water and the mobilization of resources to meet this need, major portions of the public are, apparently, poorly equipped to be self-sustaining. Therefore, current efforts to educate the public (e.g., www.ready.gov and www.prepare.gov) should be increased to encourage personal preparedness. In particular, there is a need to increase clarity about expected duration of outages and the amounts of water that individuals should maintain (e.g., 1 gallon per person per day). Consideration should be given to a strategy that leverages private industry for public service announcements and advertising to elevate this message. The Consumer Confidence Report (annual water quality reports provided to consumers pursuant to the Consumer Confidence Report Rule, 63 Fed. Reg. 44511 (Aug. 19, 1998), published at 40 C.F.R. Part 141 Subpart O) may be a useful vehicle for targeted communication on the need for personal preparedness.

Finding VIII - Develop strategies to improve the efficiency of providing an emergency water supply.

Conduct Timeline Analysis – In order to determine what items would benefit from strategy refinement, it would be useful to conduct a timeline analysis on the provision of potable water. The analysis should include various sources (e.g., local, commercial, Corps), amounts required, transportation to potentially affected areas for the affected population, and duration of maximum credible events. It should also include the time from the event to assessment of damages, requests for assistance, locating existing resources, obtaining approvals, transportation issues, mobilization of production lines for additional equipment, site set-up, security, staffing, monitoring, etc.

Foster Innovative Responses – Assess plausible innovative response strategies that can be considered for further development and application in major disaster scenarios (see Appendix B).

- The feasibility of the provision of emergency water supplies using bottled water should be evaluated in terms of procurement, supply, capacity, transport, and distribution to individuals.
- Alternative drinking water strategies should be considered in settings where there is significant risk that an imported bottled water strategy would be insufficient. For example, in some less-developed countries, approaches have included household treatment, disseminated treatment, developing temporary distribution systems, or even re-location of people for greater proximity to water and shelter (WHO 2002).[19] Relevant federal grant programs could be used to stimulate innovation along these lines (e.g., scaling up mobile package treatment units, decentralized treatment strategies, provisional distribution systems).
- Supplementing bottled water with containerized units for bulk water production should be examined as a strategy. Note that the largest units currently available have maximum unit capacity of 1 million gallon per day and little inventory of such containerized units currently exists.

---

[18] Recent analysis of the consequence of a Sacramento levee failure indicated that up to 25 million people could be out of drinking water. This would require 4,000 tractor trailer loads of bottled water per day for over 6 months. This is not likely a sustainable strategy (Source: USACE/FEMA 2010 Senior Leadership Seminar.)

[19] WHO 2002. See discussion on p. 95.

> **The Curious Case of Calexico**
>
> On April 4, 2010, a magnitude 7.2 earthquake hit the region around Calexico, California bordering Mexico. Among the facilities damaged were the water treatment facilities for this city of 38,000 people. In response to this damage, the City restricted water consumption to essential uses only and installed temporary treatment to compensate for damage to the reactor clarifiers. The State of California Department of Public Health was able to accelerate the approvals of the temporary treatment units and the manufacturer was able to mobilize with one week of approval. While in this case action was rapid, it was not without two notable limitations. First, even though it used a technology for potable water applications, the mobile unit was not permitted to produce for direct consumption. Treatment through the existing plant filters for potable consumption was still required because the technology was not approved for direct use by the State. Second, the scale of this application was small in comparison to the needs anticipated for a major metropolitan area.

Guide Development – During an emergency, resources are stretched and attention is thin. But significant risk issues are present, including public health, public confidence, financial, and legal issues. Developing a guide for procuring water, equipment, and associated services that addresses pre-approval of equipment, certifications, etc. is essential for a timely response. This would include:

- Developing guidance for pre-approval of alternate water supplies and portable treatment units in terms of certification, operation, monitoring, siteing and water utility system interface
- Highlighting the need for including procurement considerations in local, state and federal planning exercises
- Developing a certification database for containerized treatment units
- Developing an approved vendor database, and developing contracting strategies and pricing arrangements to allow vendors to be more responsive to fulfilling rapid mobilization (e.g., multi-year contracts, price premiums)

Interim Standards – Raise awareness of potential need, under dire circumstances, for state primacy agencies to consider issuing variances/waivers from applicable regulations (see Appendix B).

- Engage states and the Association of State Drinking Water Administrators on these issues.
- Address the potential for state-approved interim water quality standards.

Primary Role of Utility – Highlight that restoration of potable use is the top priority when water infrastructure has been compromised.

Revisit Roles – Roles and responsibilities need to be explicitly delineated during the planning process, accepted and regularly refined. It is necessary to address coordination issues including:

- Communication of emergency water supply need and coordination with FEMA starting at the regional level.
- Coordination with other agencies on issues such as transportation, staffing, crowd control, and security.

- Clarification as to who should be contacted pre- and post-event for various support functions.

10. References

ANSI/ASME-ITI/AWWA J100-10 Risk Analysis and Management for Critical Asset Protection (RAMCAP®) Standard for Risk and Resilience Management of Water and Wastewater Systems. 2010.

California. Governor's Office of Emergency Services. 2007. "Multi-Agency Response Guidance for Emergency Drinking Water Procurement & Distribution." 2nd Edition. Accessed January 14, 2011. http://www.oes.ca.gov/Operational/OESHome.nsf/PDF/Drinking%20Water%20Guidance/$file/Drink WaterGd.pdf

Connecticut. Department of Public Health. Drinking Water Section. 2008. "Bulk Water Hauling Guidelines." Revision December 18, 2007. Effective February 1, 2008. Accessed May 10, 2010. http://www.ct.gov/dph/lib/dph/drinking_water/pdf/Bulk_Water_Hauling_Guidelines.pdf

Federal Emergency Management Agency (FEMA). 2008. "Emergency Support Function #3 – Public Works and Engineering Annex." Accessed January 14, 2011. http://www.fema.gov/pdf/emergency/nrf/nrf-esf-03.pdf

Federal Emergency Management Agency. 2004. "Food and Water in an Emergency." [Pamphlet.] Federal Emergency Management Agency and American Red Cross. FEMA 477 A5055. http://www.fema.gov/pdf/library/f&web.pdf

Federal Emergency Management Agency. 2003. "Emergency Support Function #8 – Health and Medical Services Annex." Accessed January 14, 2011. http://www.fema.gov/pdf/emergency/nrf/nrf-esf-08.pdf

New Jersey. Department of Environmental Protection. 2007. "Interconnection Study Mitigation of Water Supply Emergencies – Public Version." Prepared by Gannett Fleming, and Black and Veatch.

Oxfam. 2010. Water and Sanitation. Maintaining Standards. [Web page] Accessed February 10, 2011. http://www.oxfam.org.uk/oxfam_in_action/emergencies/whatwedo/watsan.html

R.A. Reed and R.J. Shaw. 1999. Emergency water supply. [Well technical brief #44]. In "Running Water." Ed. R. Shaw. London: Water, Engineering and Development Centre/ Intermediate Technology Publications. Accessed February 7, 2011. http://www.lboro.ac.uk/well/resources/technical-briefs/technical-briefs.htm

U.S. Army Corps of Engineers (USACE). 2006. "ESF #3 Field Guide." Accessed February 25, 2009. https://eportal.usace.army.mil/sites/ENGLink/ESF3/Shared%20Documents/ESF%203%20Field%20Gui de.pdf

U.S. Army Corps of Engineers. 1998. "Water Supply Handbook; A Handbook on Water Supply Planning and Resource Management." USACE Institute for Water Resources, Water Resource Support Center: Revised Report 96-PS-4.

U.S. Environmental Protection Agency (EPA). 2008. "Water Security Initiative: Interim Guidance on Developing Consequence Management Plans for Drinking Water Utilities." Washington, D.C.: U.S. Environmental Protection Agency, Office of Water, EPA 817-R-08-001.

U.S. Environmental Protection Agency. 2004. "Emergency Response Plan Guidance for Small and Medium Community Water Systems to Comply with the Public Health Security and Bioterrorism Preparedness and Response Act of 2002." U.S. Environmental Protection Agency, Office of Water (4601M), EPA 816-R-04-002. April 7, 2004. Accessed February 14, 2011. http://www.epa.gov/safewater/watersecurity/pubs/small_medium_ERP_guidance040704.pdf

U.S. Environmental Protection Agency. 2003. "Large Water System Emergency Response Plan Outline: Guidance to Assist Community Water Systems in Complying with the Public Health Security and Bioterrorism Preparedness and Response Act of 2002." EPA 810-F-03-007. Accessed February 5, 2009. http://www.epa.gov/safewater/watersecurity/pubs/erp-long-outline.pdf

U.S. Department of Homeland Security. 2009. "Ready.gov – Prepare. Plan. Stay Informed." Accessed January 14, 2011. http://www.ready.gov/

World Health Organization (WHO). 2005. "Cleaning and disinfecting water storage tanks and tankers." Technical Notes for Emergencies, Technical Note No. 3. Revised July 1, 2005. Accessed May 10, 2010. http://www.searo.who.int/LinkFiles/List_of_Guidelines_for_Health_Emergency_Cleaning_and_disinfecting_water_storage_tanks.pdf

WHO. 2002. "Environmental health in emergencies and disasters: a practical guide." Edited by B. Wisner and J. Adams. Geneva, Switzerland: World Health Organization. Accessed March 1, 2011. http://www.who.int/water_sanitation_health/hygiene/emergencies/emergencies2002/en/

Appendix A – Post-Disaster Water Supply: Haiti and Other International Disasters – What Can We Learn About Scale-Up for Water Provision?

On June 17, 2010, a panel was assembled in Washington, D.C. to reflect on the relevance of previous international disasters to potential response to a catastrophic disaster in the United States. The agenda consisted of the following:

1. Objectives
2. Background
3. Scenarios of Concern
4. Reflections on Various Case Studies
5. Key Issues
6. Recommendations

Objectives

Gather insight from international experience with post-incident water provisioning to determine what lessons can be extrapolated to U.S. domestic planning efforts to develop an effective catastrophic disaster assistance approach. This includes policy, institutional, and logistical issues in providing an emergency water supply (e.g., procurement, transportation, ancillary equipment, security) along with lessons learned on rate-limiting steps in implementation.

Issues for Consideration

Several key findings were articulated by the participants for improving response to catastrophic disasters:

1. *Streamlining and improving quality of information management* – Experience has underscored the challenge to develop accurate situational awareness for good decision making. Much data gathering occurs after a disaster, but the gathering is often uncoordinated and the data is of varying quality. In addition, poor data analysis can lead to inaccurate understanding of the actual situation. There is a significant need for improving coordination of data collection; systematic and robust analysis of pooled data; review of findings; and concise summaries of the information portraying the situation to decision makers, the press, and other stakeholders.

2. *Greater adherence to the Incident Command System (ICS) model* – A major factor inhibiting an effective, streamlined response after a catastrophic disaster is the sheer number of entities that are involved: political (local, regional, national and international), technical, operational, administrative, NGOs, random volunteers, etc. The frequency and duration of the meetings to inform various political and managerial levels can divert key personnel from the response. The participants affirmed the benefit of the ICS model in maintaining clear lines of control and accountability for disaster management, and they noted that it streamlines policy considerations that could otherwise slow and inhibit a response. Coordination and communication between

major players is essential. It helps to limit conflicts of jurisdiction, overlapping responses, and underutilized resources that could delay effective responses.

3. *Setting expectations early* –After a catastrophic disaster, assistance may take more than a week to become fully operational. Public education that emphasizes personal preparedness is needed, particularly for those living in areas most vulnerable to disaster. Examples of public education include the Federal Emergency Management Agency (FEMA)'s READY.gov program or the joint FEMA/American Red Cross campaign. Greater levels of resilience at the individual level will significantly mitigate demands on response and recovery efforts.

4. *Developing more creative approaches to post-catastrophe response* – There was a shared recognition that traditional approaches may not work after a catastrophic event. For example, the current approach to post-disaster water supply in the United States is bottled water. The logistics and sustainability of such an approach, however, is not feasible in a catastrophe due to the logistics of serving a multi-million person population in an urban area. More creative approaches may include developing a portfolio of emergency water supply alternatives (e.g., trucking water, large-scale and medium-scale treatment units, household purification techniques) and allowance for flexibility in administering existing regulatory requirements. It may also include more public-private partnerships to utilize existing capacity (e.g., supermarkets for water and food distribution).

5. *More fully utilizing military capabilities* – The resources of the U.S. military are significant, yet the sense of some participants was that the military has not been used effectively in many response efforts. More thought as to pre-determined roles and tasks for military could enhance effectiveness of response significantly. The greatest emphasis in enhancing response effectiveness should be on logistical support, not on command/control issues.

6. *Remembering that sanitation and hygiene are critical to public health protection* – While the discussions were focused on water provision, the 2010 Haiti earthquake experience highlights the importance of maintaining adequate sanitation and hygiene to protect the public health.

Appendix B: Interim Water Quality Targets

This workshop held in Washington, D.C. on January 28, 2010 assembled experts from NGOs, local, state and federal agencies to consider emergency water supplies and to brainstorm potential strategies for improving the effectiveness of the response. The agenda consisted of several items:

1. Objectives
2. Background
   - Emergency water plan
   - Limiters on response
   - Stakeholder issues
3. Potential circumstances that could trigger need
4. Precedents
   - Tri-service standards
   - Environmental Protection Agency (EPA) Protective Action Guides
   - World Health Organization standards
   - Prior disasters
   - Other
5. Scenarios
6. Key Issues
7. Recommendations

Objectives

This workshop was prompted by the specter of a disaster of unprecedented scale for the U.S. that would trigger a severely time-limited, resource-constrained response to acute public health needs. More specifically, during three 2009 workshops which focused on supplying potable water after a major disaster, participants from local, regional, state and federal government agencies, as well as the private sector, all asked whether relief from some regulatory requirements – referred to as "interim standards" – would be possible post-disaster as this might improve the timeliness of providing water.

Conclusions

Four principal conclusions were drawn:

1. An epic catastrophe impacting a region with millions of people would increase a multiplicity of public health risks.
2. The recovery period would likely be of a long duration since events that impact drinking water systems also have profound primary impacts on other infrastructure (e.g., power, transportation, communications) and secondary impacts (e.g., disruption to supply chains, mobility difficulties, security concerns, human-resource depletion).
3. There is precedent, and likely a need during emergencies, for adjusting water-quality goals during the recovery period.[20]

---

[20] Variance and exemptions from certain regulatory provisions may be granted in accordance with 40 C.F.R. § 141.4(a). The authority to grant variances or exemptions confers as part of state primacy with EPA oversight.

4. Supporting scientific information is available to assist utilities and states in formulating a recovery strategy.

Issues for Consideration

A number of action items were formulated by the panel for further consideration:

1. *Form a Strike team to assist in decision-making*: Building on existing resources (e.g., the Federal-State Toxicology and Risk Analysis Committee, health advisory (HA) database,[21] and the red team of EPA's National Homeland Security Research Center), develop a strike team to assist those making judgments as to interim regulatory requirements.

2. *Database assessment and augmentation*: Perform a data gap analysis and expand the number of health advisories and numeric recommendations based on what is available in existing resources (i.e., the U.S. Department of Defense Chemical, Biological, Radiological and Nuclear Defense Information Analysis Center; the U.S. EPA Integrated Risk Information System; the Occupational Safety and Health Administration's listing of Permissible Exposure Levels).[22] In order to inform the gap analysis: (a) elicit local-state feedback on which contaminants could raise concerns during a natural major disaster, (b) promote and support local-state tabletop emergency response exercises on risk-balancing scenarios, and (c) encourage feedback to EPA on information gaps and challenges.

3. *Develop a contaminant treatment technology testing, certification, and verification database for use by states:* Consider developing a 3-tiered certification system based on basic containerized treatment systems (e.g., pathogen removal, inactivation, select contaminant removal) plus energy requirements, residuals production, costs, and operational requirements.[23]

4. *Provide guidance on risk communication*: Since it is critical to involve risk communication specialists early in any situation that would entail provisional risk-balancing, guidance on risk communication should be accessible at state and local levels.[24]

---

[21] EPA Drinking Water Health Advisories Tables
http://water.epa.gov/action/advisories/drinking/drinking_index.cfm#dw-standards

[22] CBRNIAC https://www.cbrniac.apgea.army.mil/About/InformationResources/Pages/default.aspx; IRIS http://www.epa.gov/iris/, drinking water health advisories http://www.epa.gov/waterscience/criteria/drinking/#dw-standards, OSHA PELs (Permissible Exposure Levels) http://www.osha.gov/SLTC/pel/, FASTRAC (Federal and State Toxicology and Risk Assessment Committee) http://www.epa.gov/waterscience/fstrac/intro.html, and CSAC (Chemical Security Analysis Center http://www.dhs.gov/files/labs/gc_1225399127004.shtm. DOD resources include ftp://ftp.rta.nato.int/PubFullText/RTO/MP/RTO-MP-HFM-086/MP-HFM-086-11.pdf http://chppm-www.apgea.army.mil/dehe/pgm31/WaterRef.aspx

[23] See ETV http://www.epa.gov/etv/ and NSF http://www.nsf.org/business/drinking_water_systems_center/index.asp?program=DrinkingWatSysCen http://www.nsf.org/business/water_distribution/index.asp?program=WaterDistributionSys

[24] CDC's *Guide to Drinking Water Advisories* will be released in spring 2011, it presents protocols for utilities and agencies to address situations that generate either system- or state-initiated advisories. .

---

5. *Train state-level public-health decision-makers:* Decision-makers should become aware of the health risk information available, its limitations, and its applicability to decisions concerning acute and long-term health risks arising from disasters.

6. *Educate the public on the need for personal preparedness including other measures that have multiple benefits*: Use existing programs such as www.ready.gov and other means to educate the public on personal preparedness.

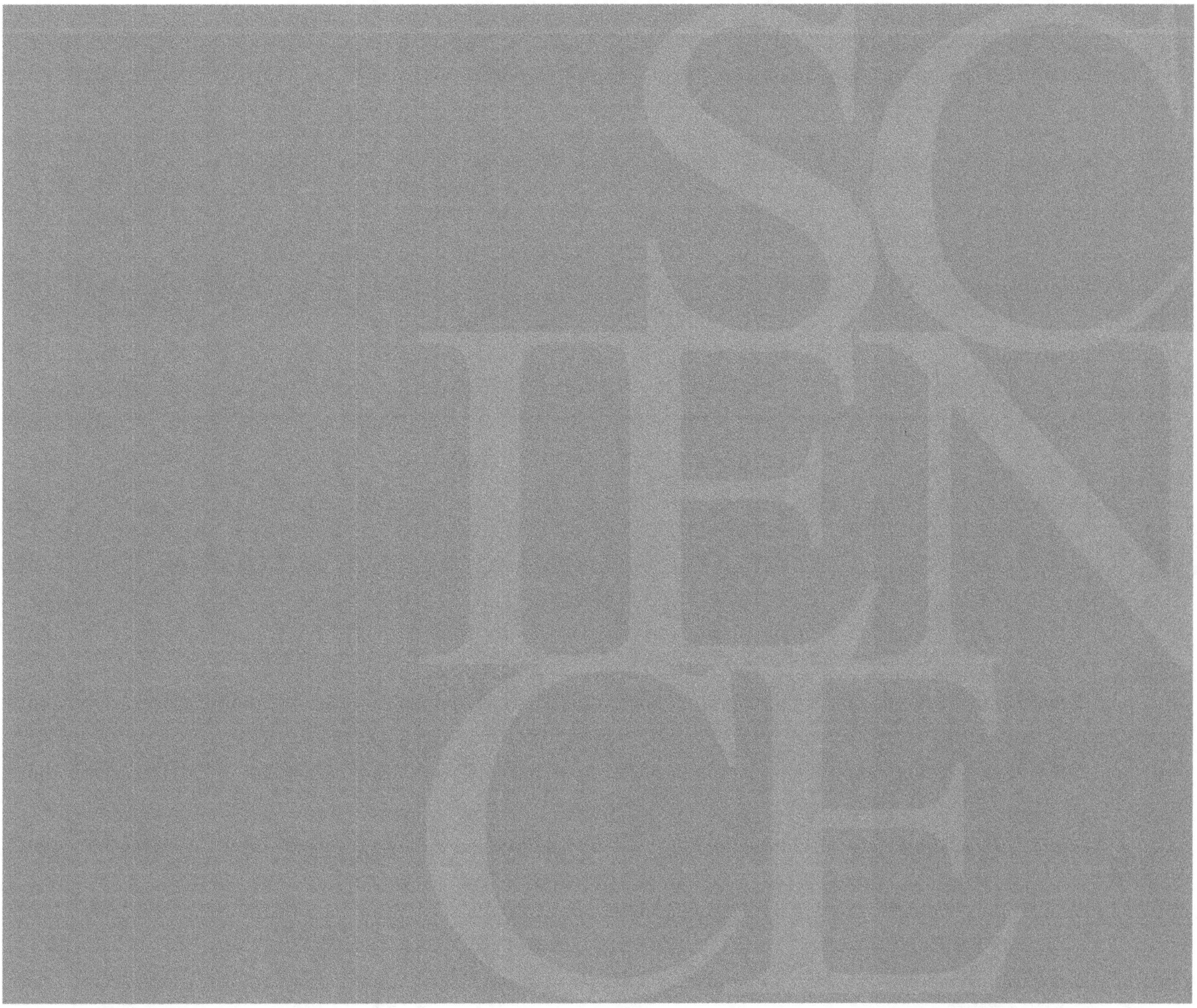

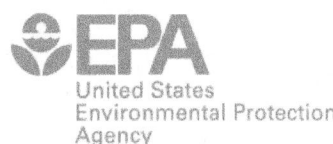
United States
Environmental Protection
Agency

Office of Research and Development (8101R)
Washington, DC 20460

www.ingramcontent.com/pod-product-compliance
Lightning Source LLC
Chambersburg PA
CBHW081905170526
45167CB00007B/3161